Neuroanatomy

COLORING BOOK

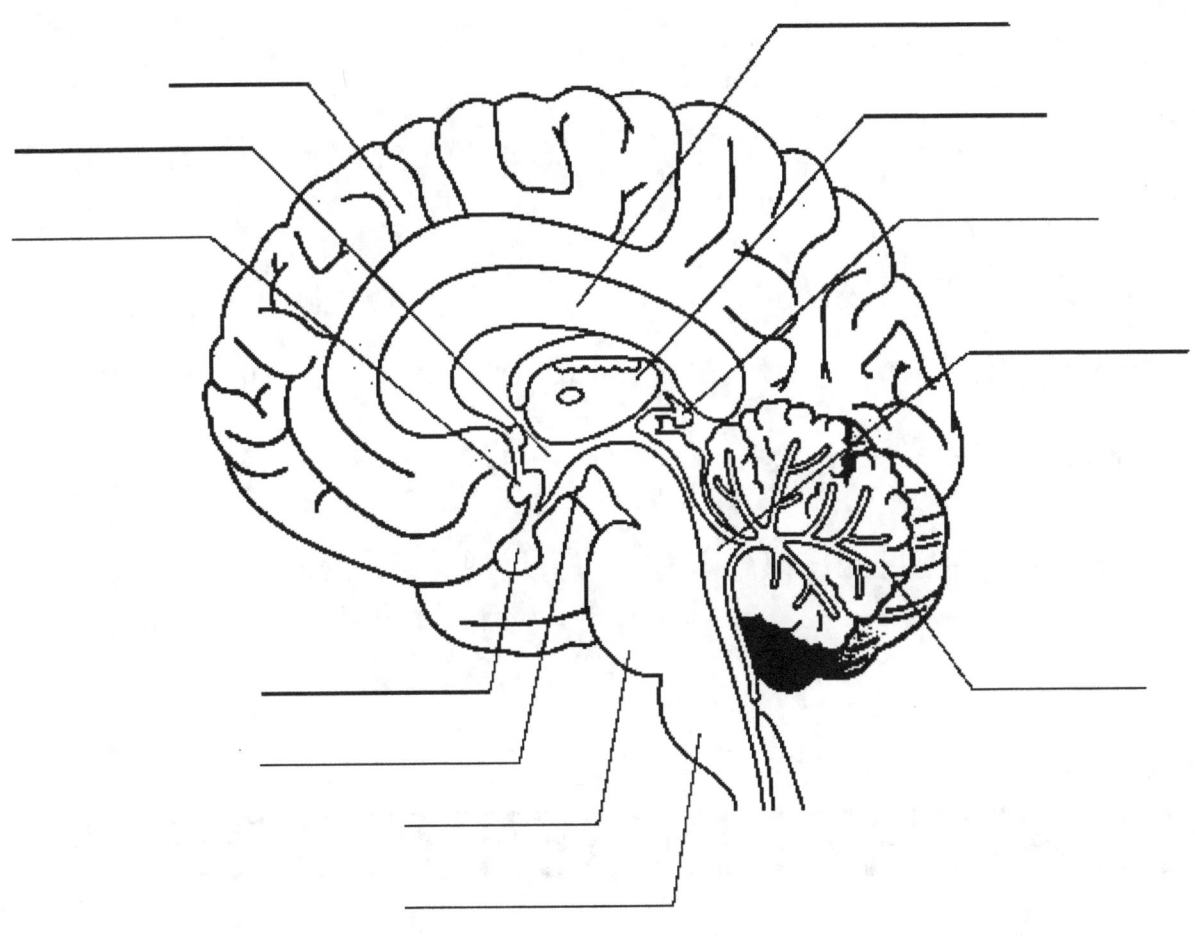

THIS BOOK BELONG TO :

_____

_____

These Illustrations Show The Brain And Its Components And Makes It Easy To Identify Specific Structures For An Entertaining Way To Learn Neuroanatomy.

ALL RIGHTS RESERVED 2024:

COLOR TEST

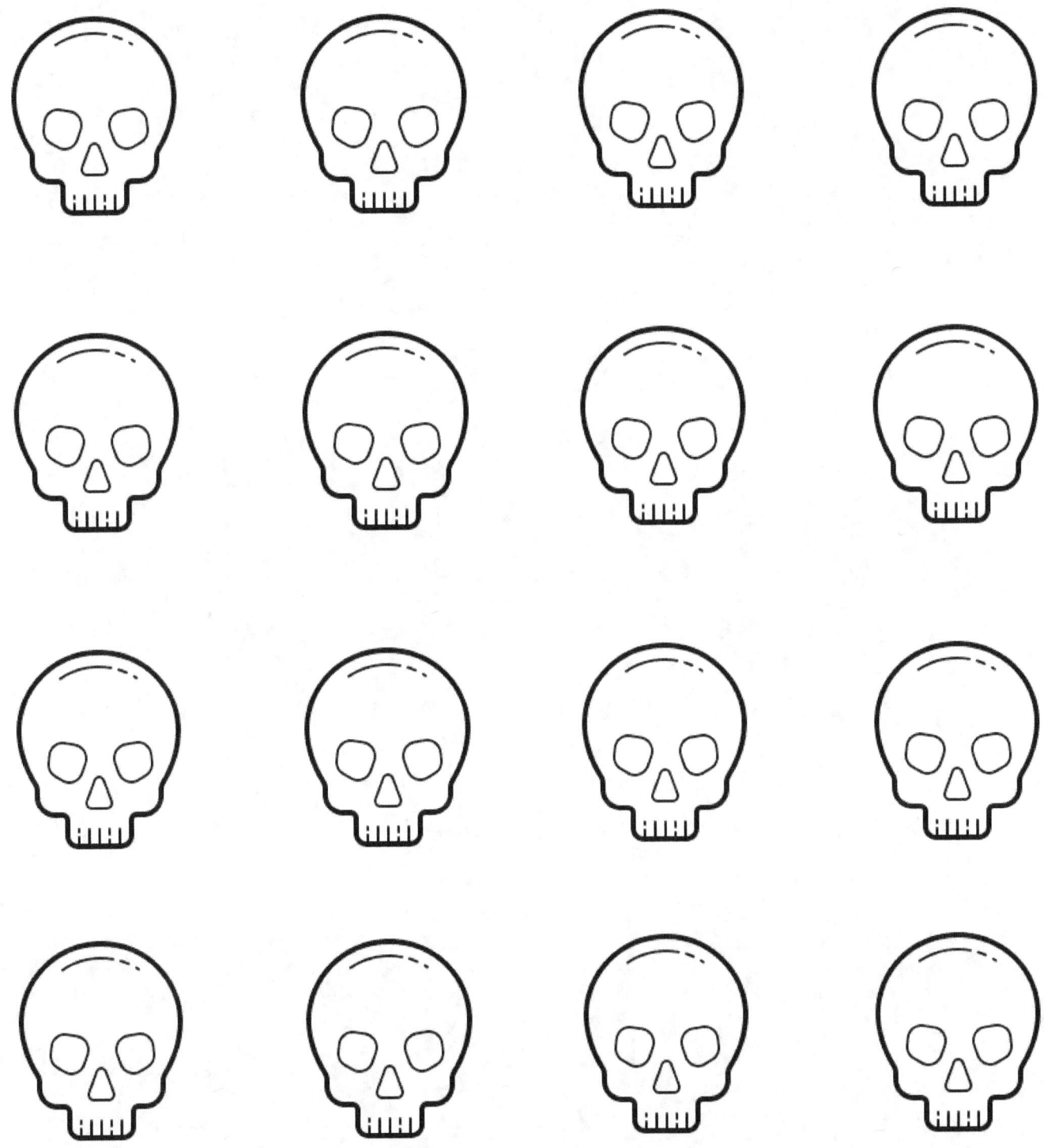

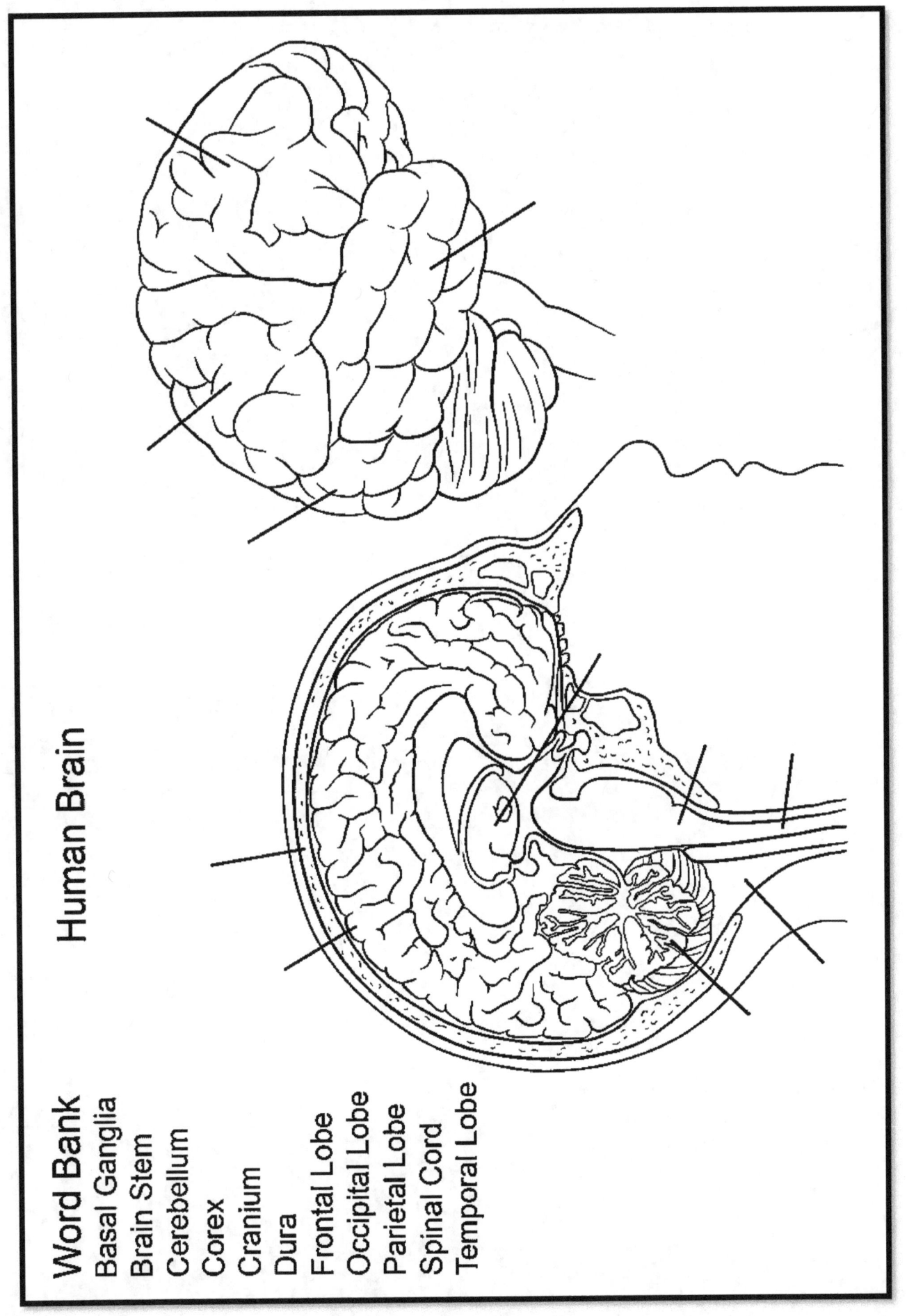

Human Brain

Word Bank
Basal Ganglia
Brain Stem
Cerebellum
Corex
Cranium
Dura
Frontal Lobe
Occipital Lobe
Parietal Lobe
Spinal Cord
Temporal Lobe

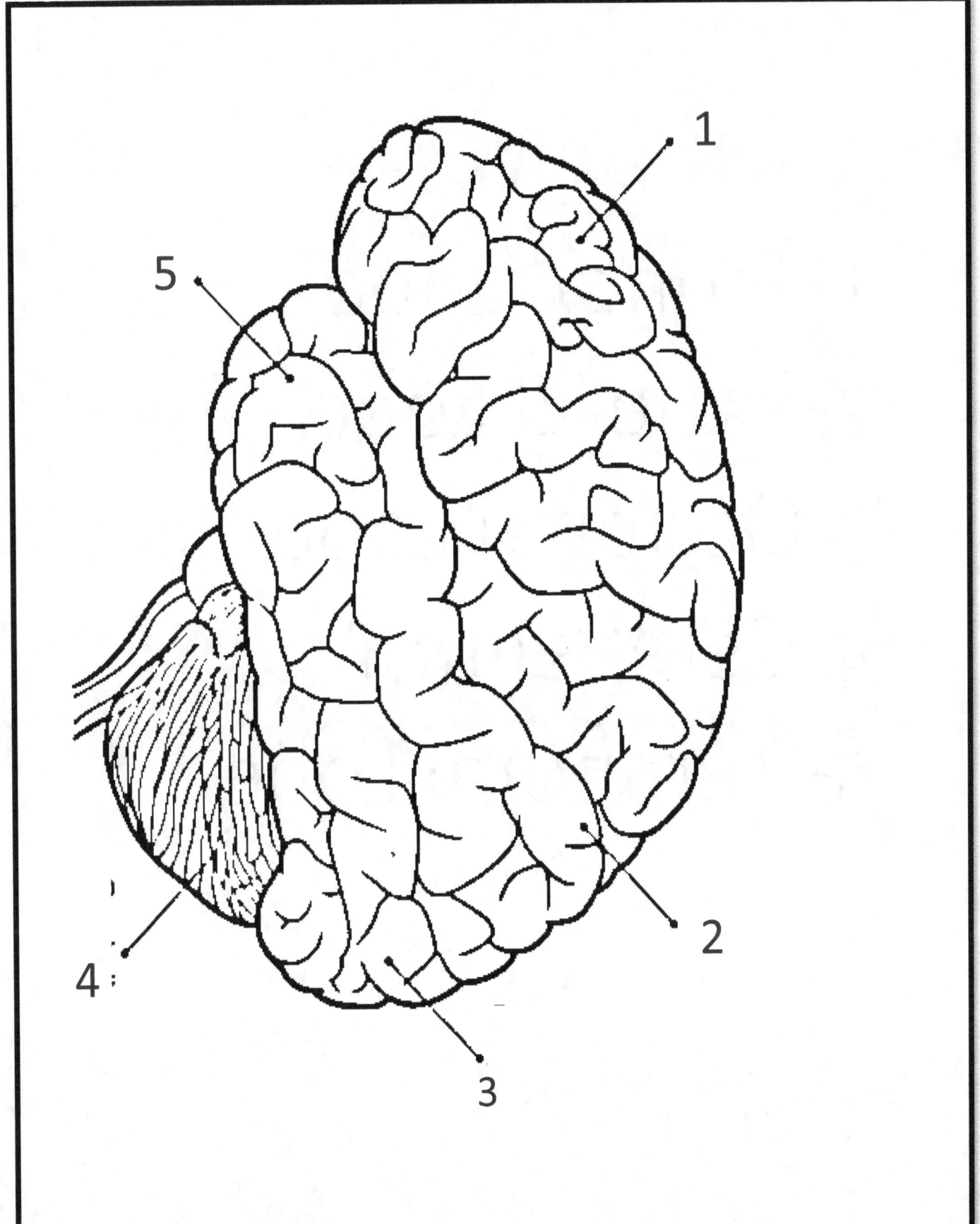

1

5

4

3

2

1- Frontal Lobe

2-Parietal Lobe

3-Occipital Lobe

4-Cerebellum

5- Temporal Lobe

FUNCTIONAL AREAS OF THE BRAIN

LATERAL VIEW

PARIETAL LOBE

FRONTAL LOBE

OCCIPITAL LOBE

TEMPORAL LOBE

CEREBELLUM

BRAIN STEM

SHOWS THE THREE MAJOR CORRIDOR OF THE BRAIN. THESE ARE THE MIND, CEREBELLUM AND BRAINSTEM

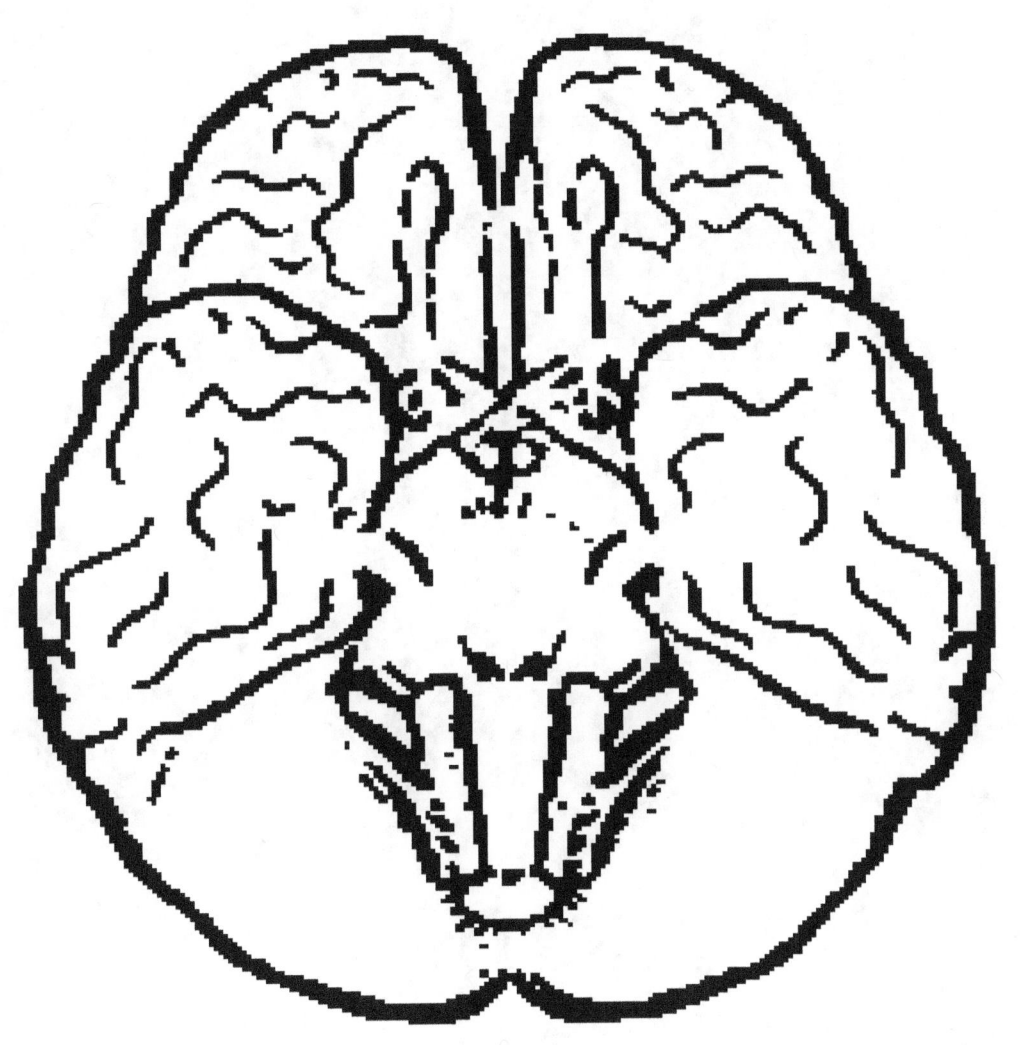

INFERIOR VIEW

divides the right and left side

of the brain into corridor

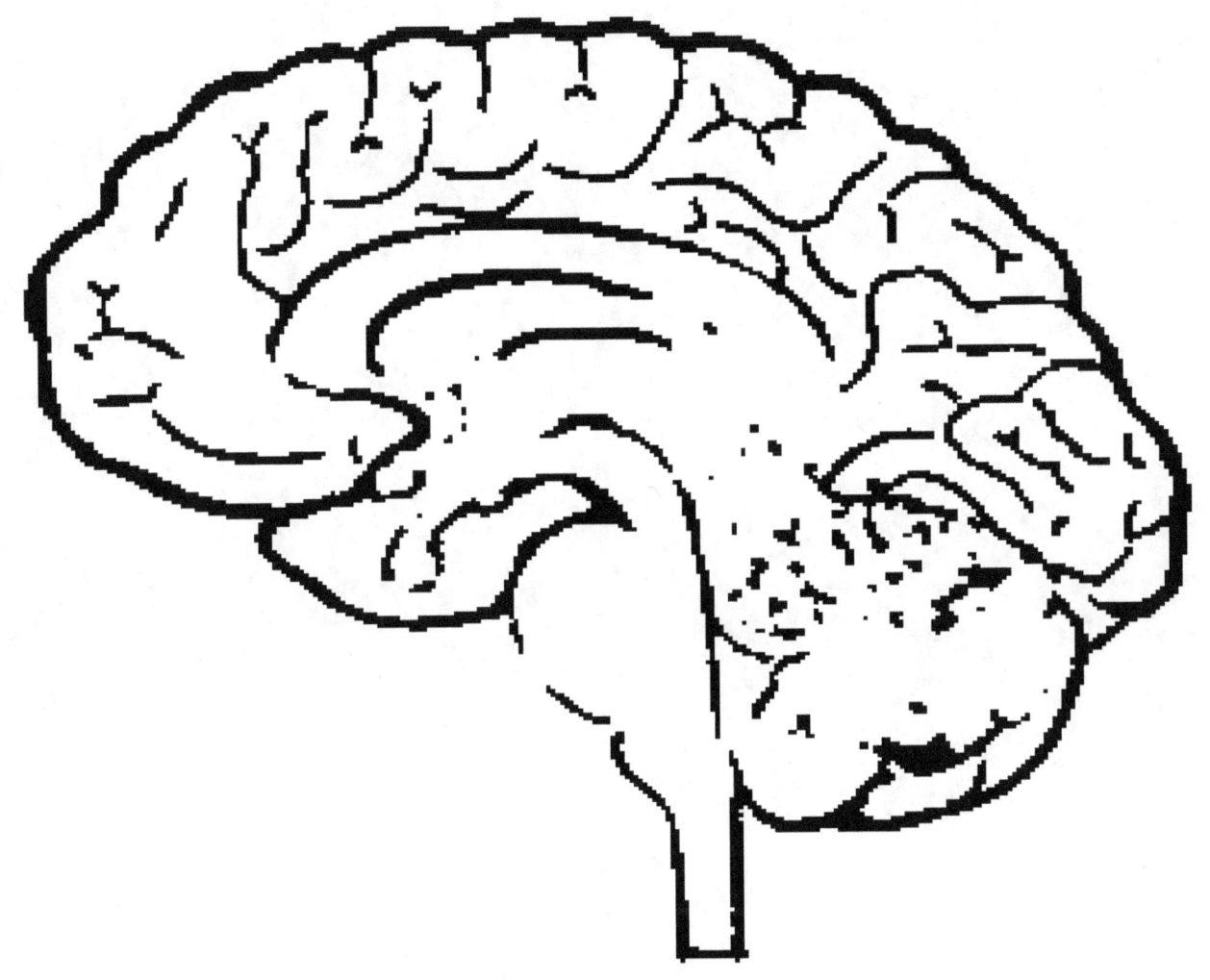

SAGITTAL VIEW

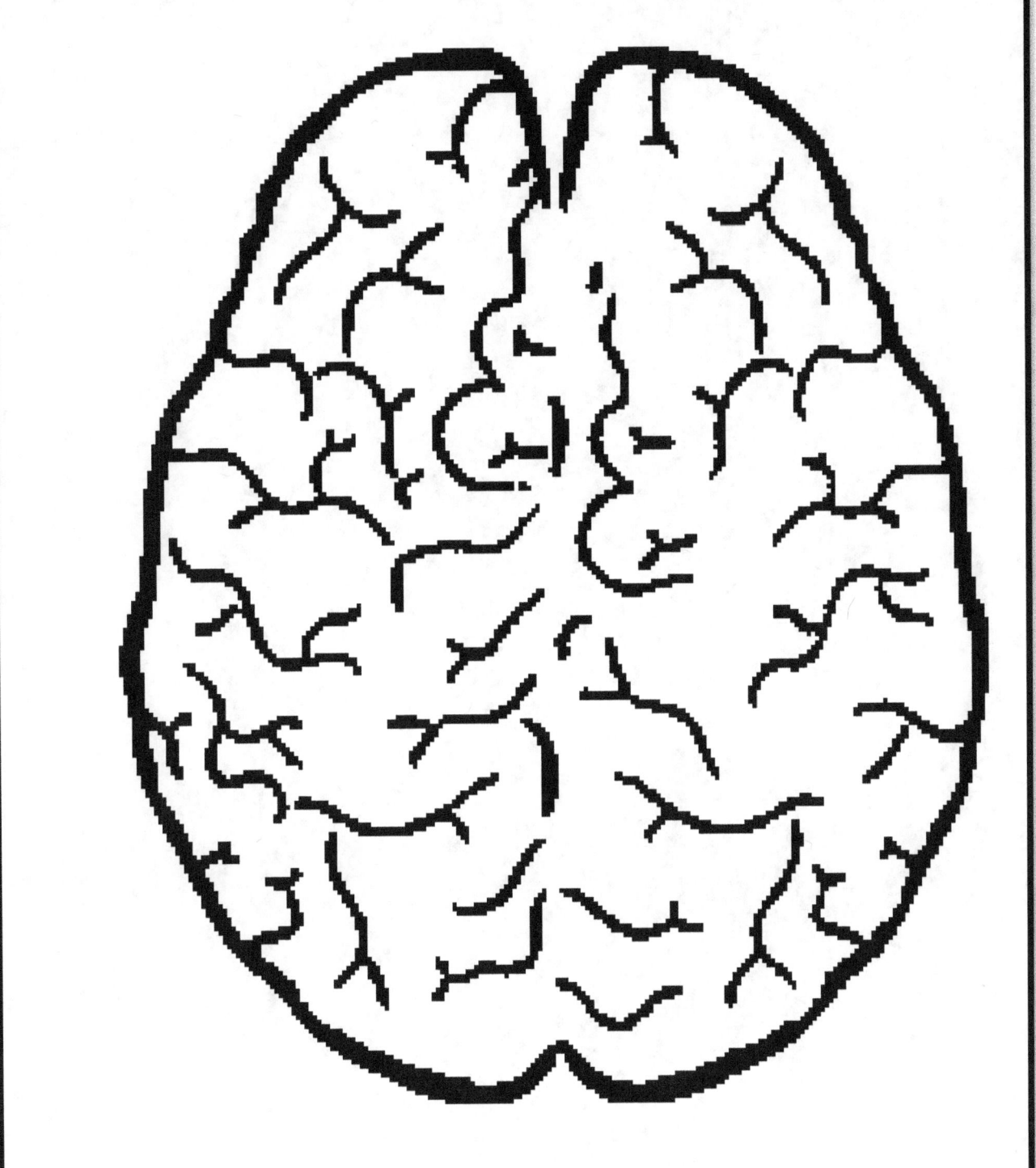

SUPERIOR VIEW

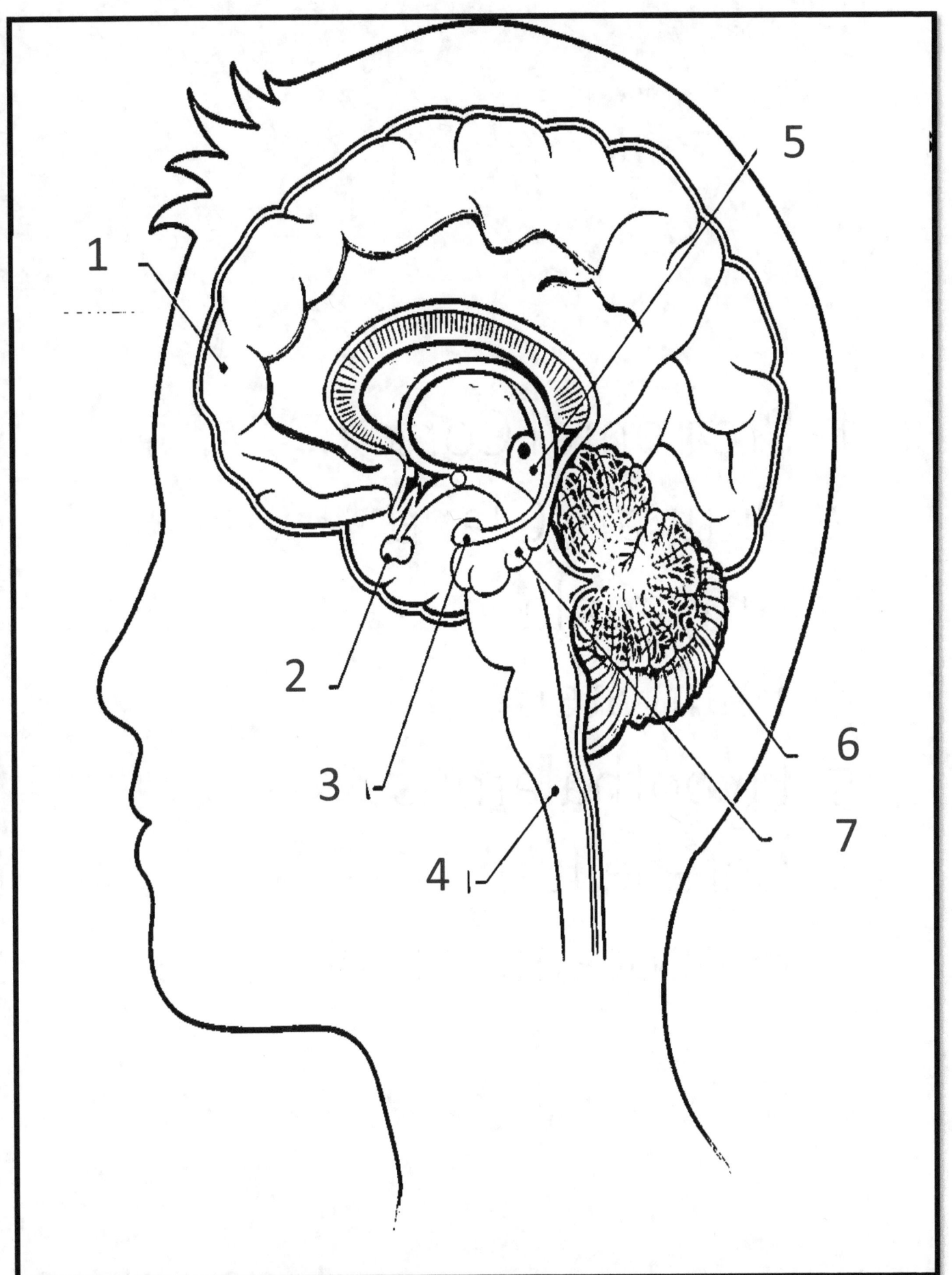

17

1- Prefrontal Cortex

2- Pituitary Gland

3- Amygdala

4- Brain Stem

5- Hypothalamus

6- Cerebellum

7- Hippocampus

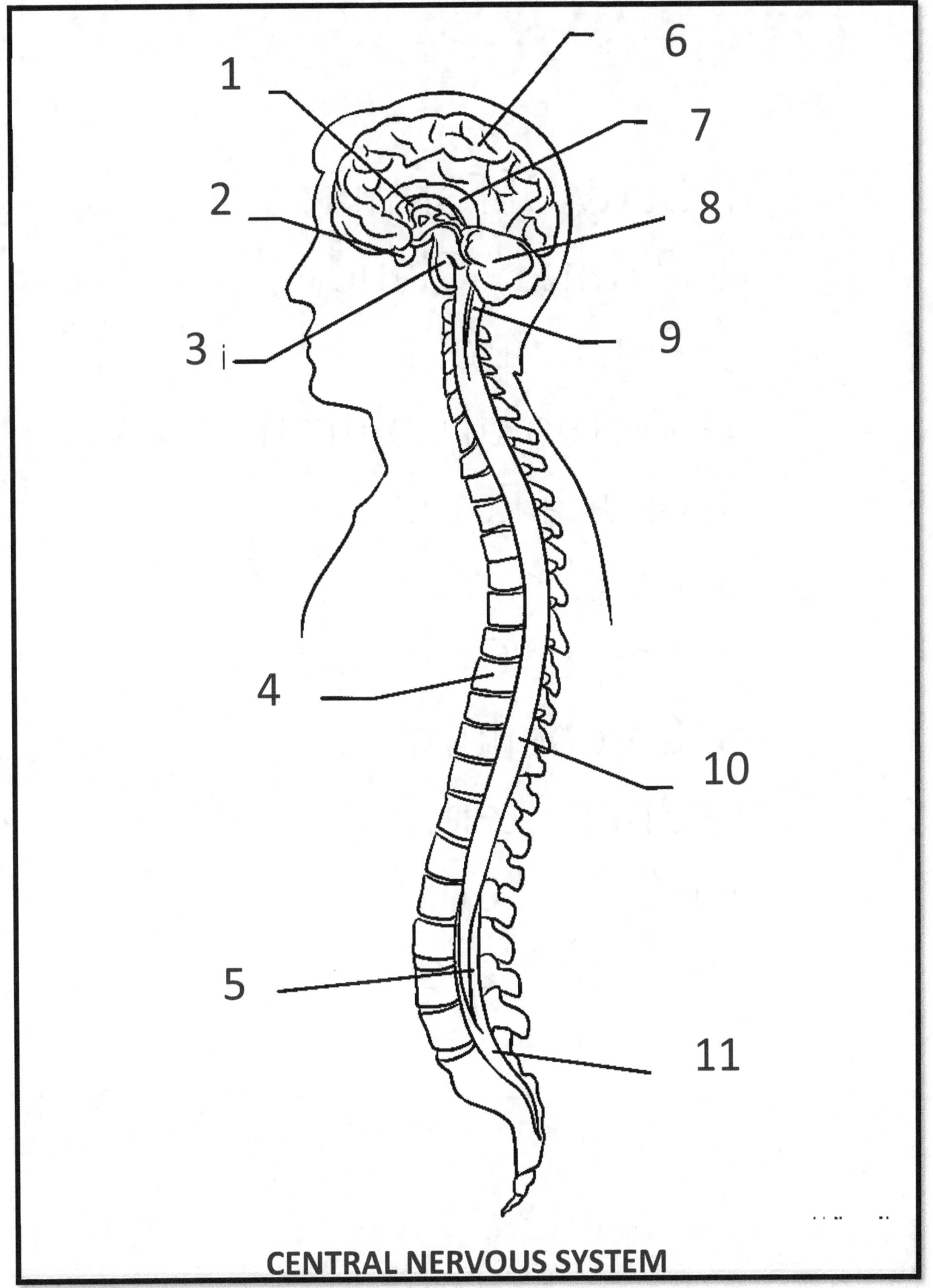

CENTRAL NERVOUS SYSTEM

1- Body Of Formix

2- Pituitary Gland

3- Pons Varolii

4- Vertebral Column

5- Cauda Equina

6- Cerebrum

7- Corpus Callosum

8- Cerebellum

9- Brain Stem

10- Spinal Cord

11- Dura Mater

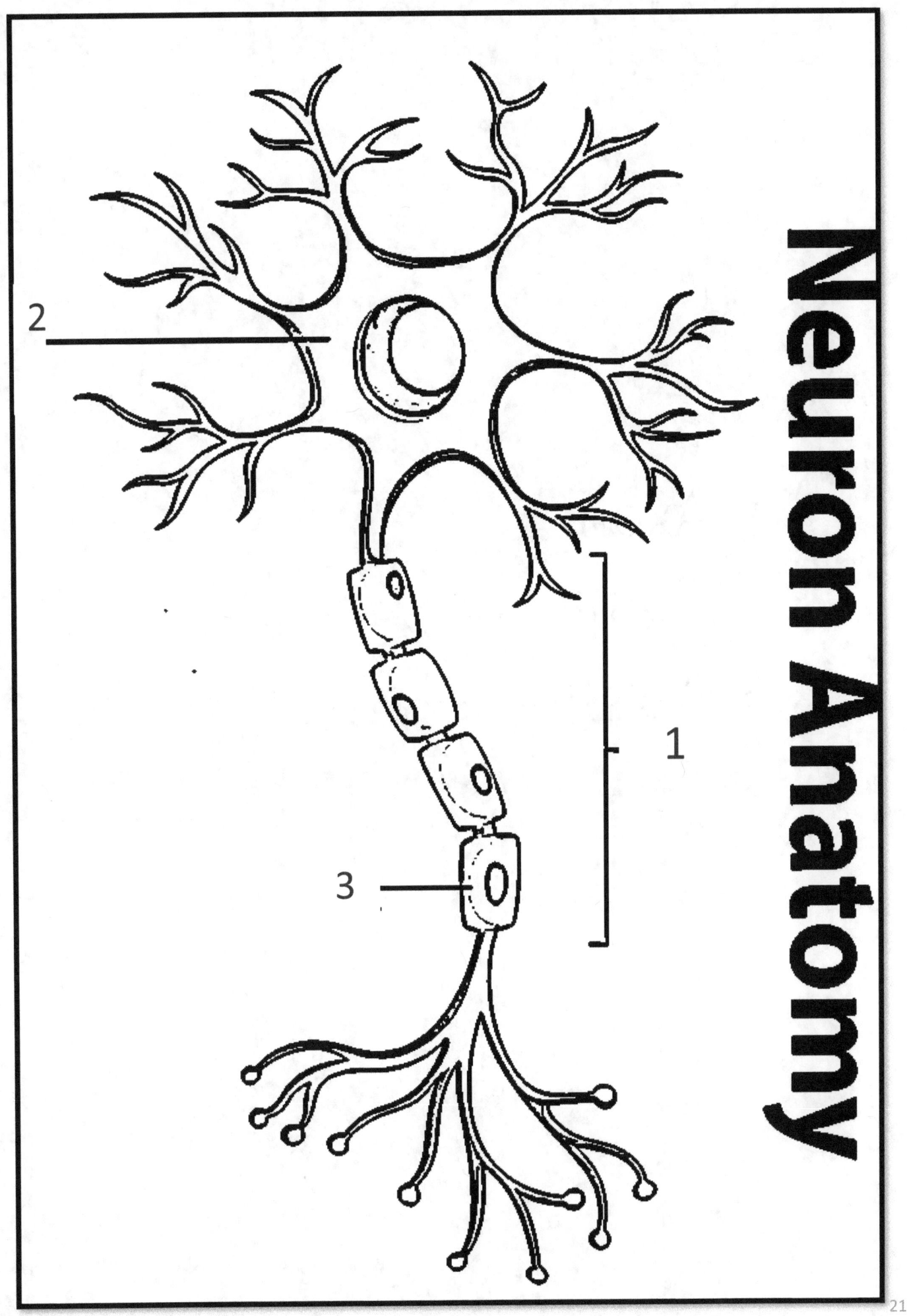

2 _____

1

3 ———

Neuron Anatomy

1- Axon

2- Soma

3- Myelin

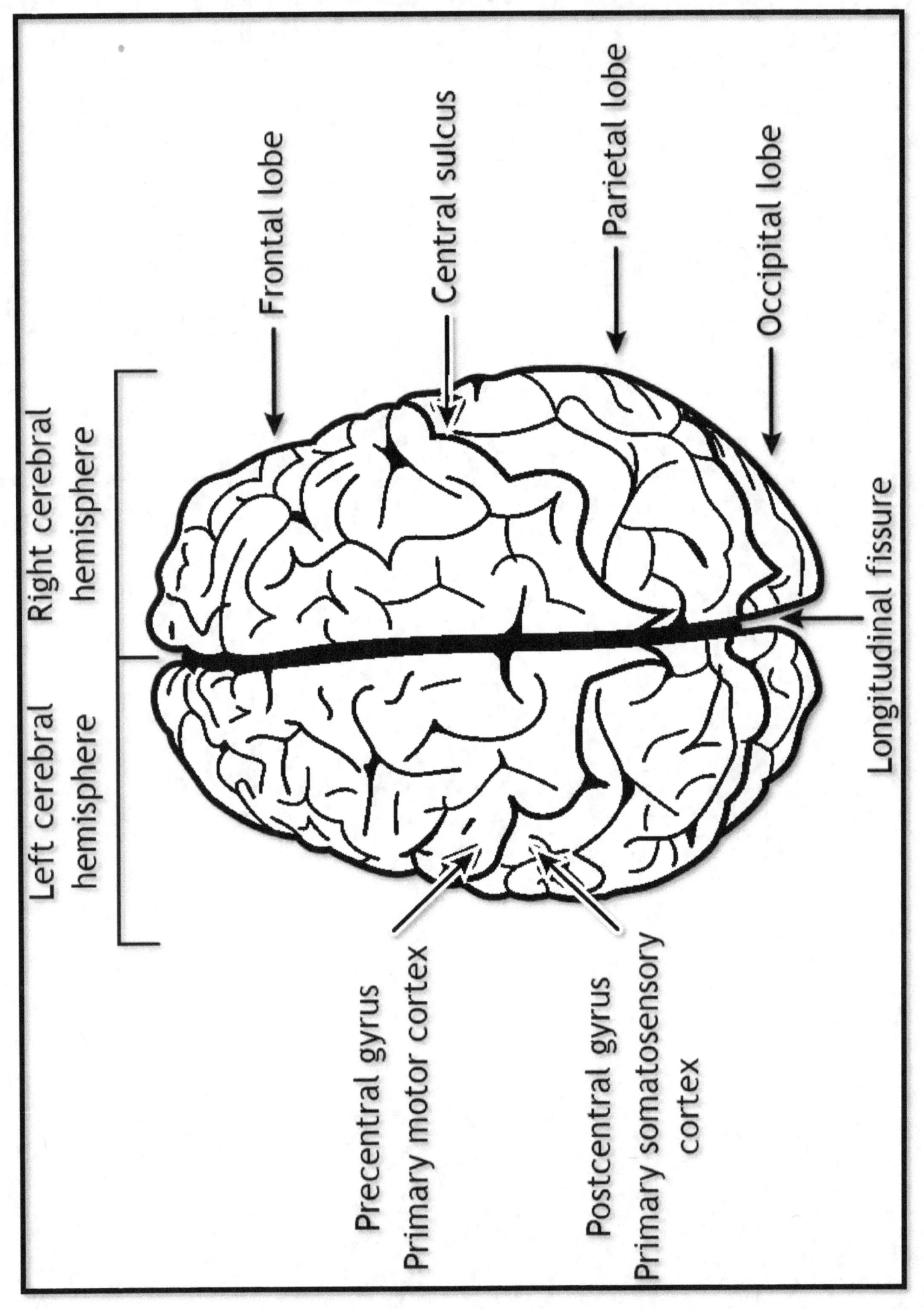

Frontal lobe

Central sulcus

Parietal lobe

Occipital lobe

Longitudinal fissure

Right cerebral hemisphere

Left cerebral hemisphere

Precentral gyrus
Primary motor cortex

Postcentral gyrus
Primary somatosensory cortex

LIMBIC SYSTEM

Interthalamic adhesion

Corpus callosum

Fornix

Thalamus

Occipital lobe

Cingulate gyrus

Cerebellum

Choroid plexus

Anterior group of thalamic nuclei

Frontal lobe

Cingulate gyrus

Hypothalamus

Amygdala

Mamillary body

Hippocampus

Brain stem

BRAIN STEM

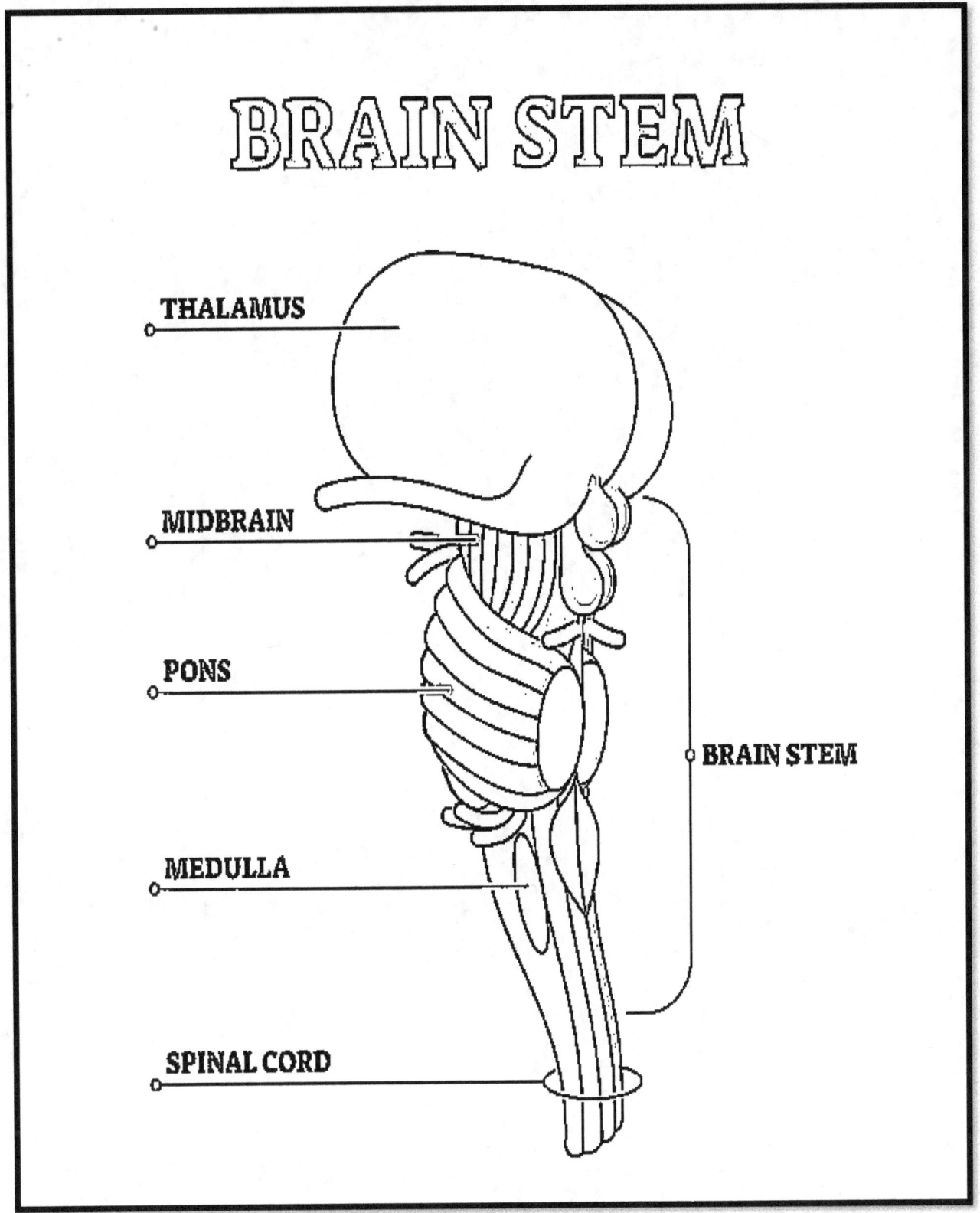

THALAMUS

MIDBRAIN

PONS

BRAIN STEM

MEDULLA

SPINAL CORD

AREA AT THE BASE OF THE BRAIN THAT LIES BETWEEN THE DEEP STRUCTURES OF THE CEREBRAL COMPONENTS AND THE CERVICAL SPINAL CORD AND THAT SERVES A CRITICAL PART IN REGULATING CERTAIN INVOLUNTARY CONDUCT OF THE BODY, INCLUDING TWINKLE AND BREATHING

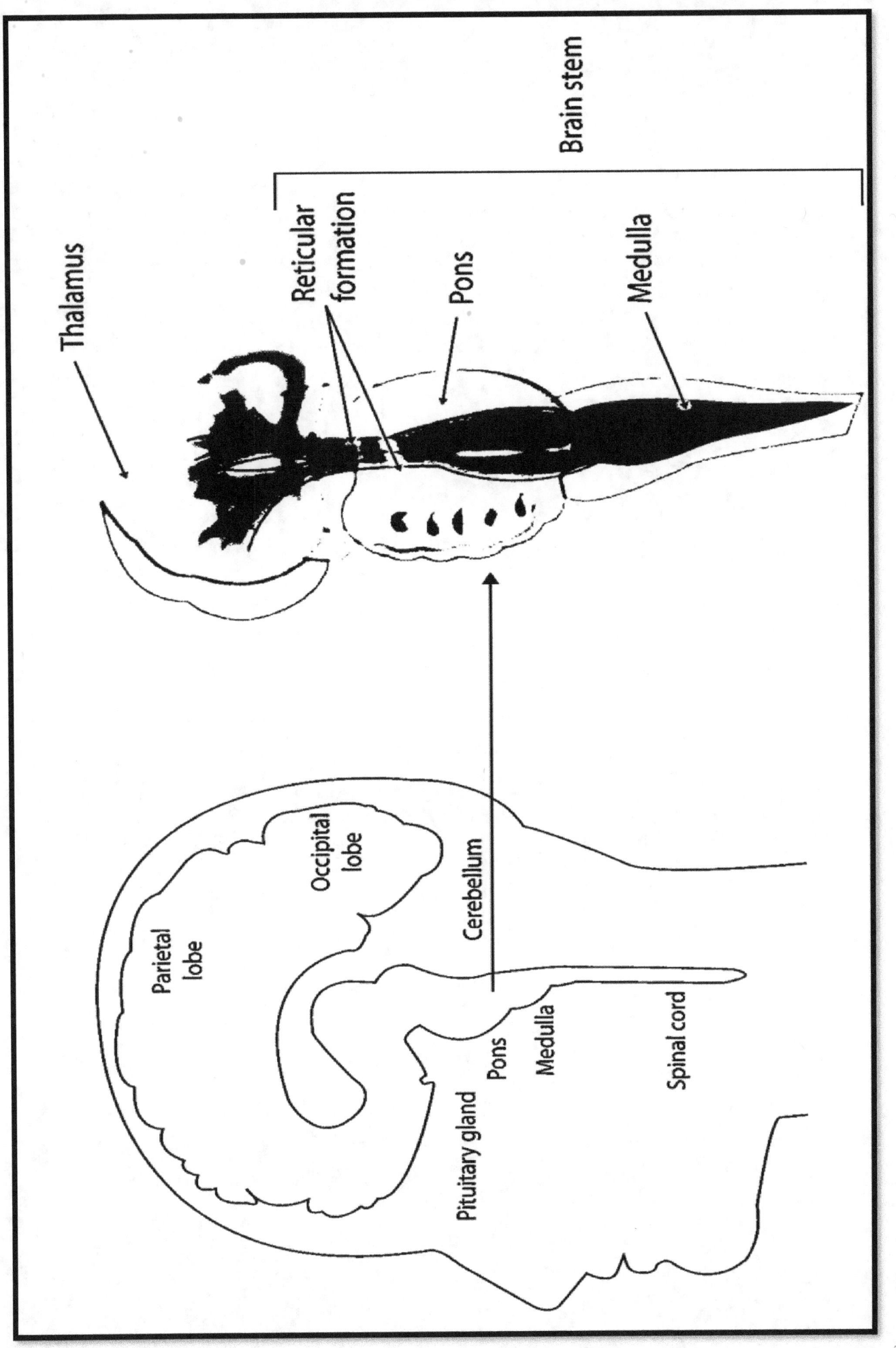

Thalamus

Reticular formation

Pons

Medulla

Brain stem

Parietal lobe

Occipital lobe

Cerebellum

Pituitary gland

Pons

Medulla

Spinal cord

Serotonin pathway

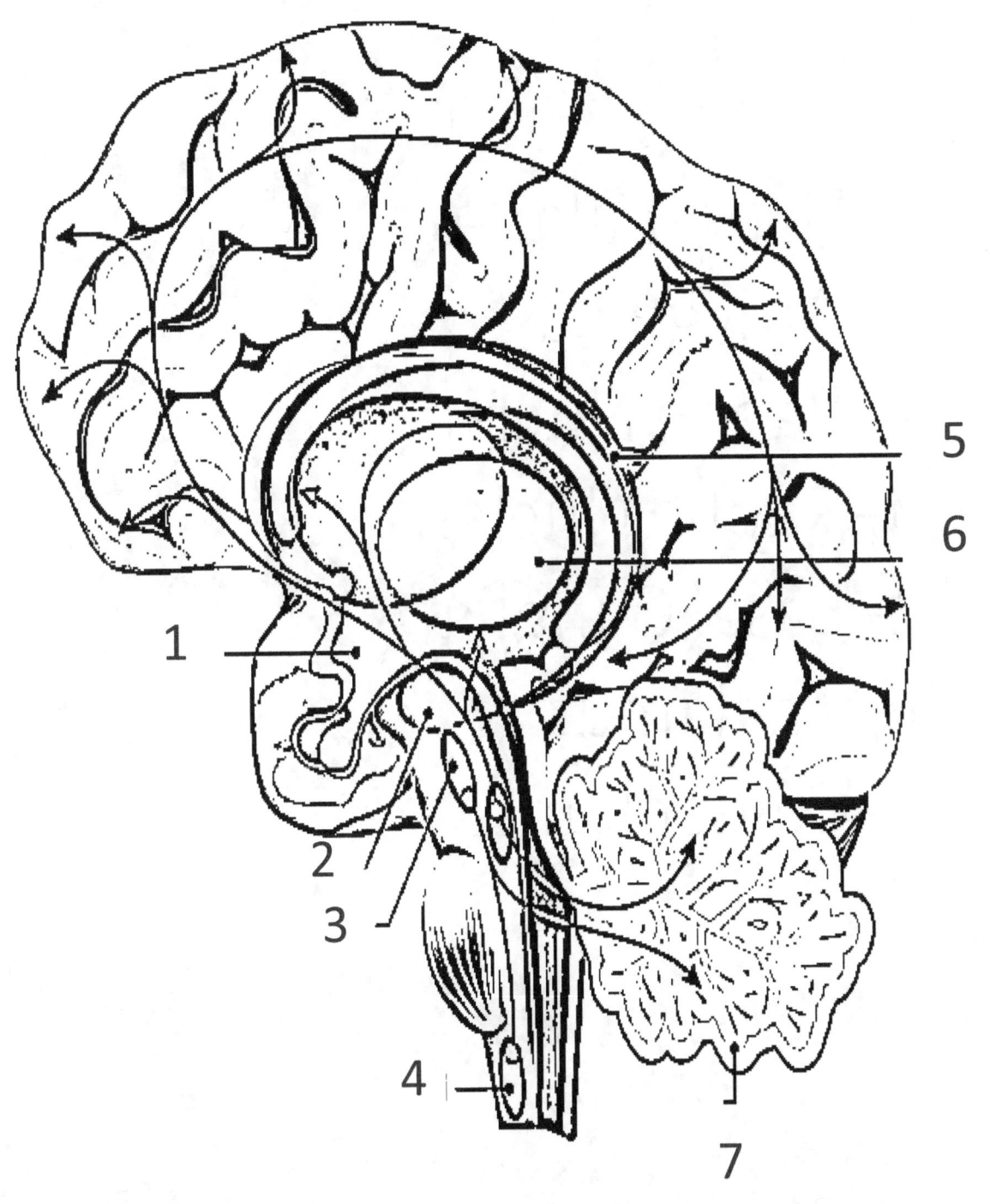

1- Hypothalamus
2- Amygdala
3- Raphe Nuclei
4- Raphe Nuclei
5- Basal Ganglia
6- Thalamus
7- Cerebellum

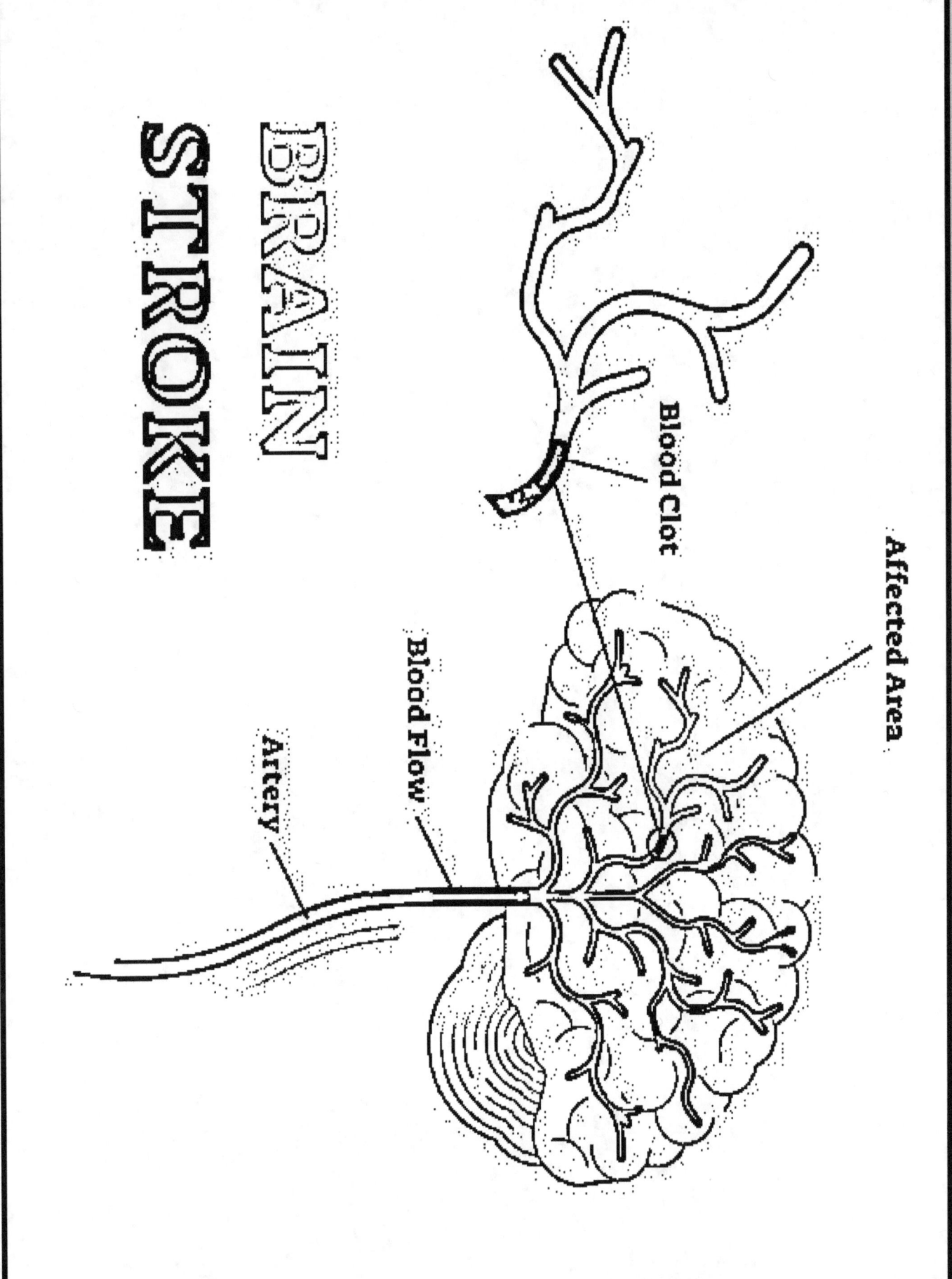

BRAIN STROKE

Blood Clot

Affected Area

Blood Flow

Artery

BRAIN STIMULATION

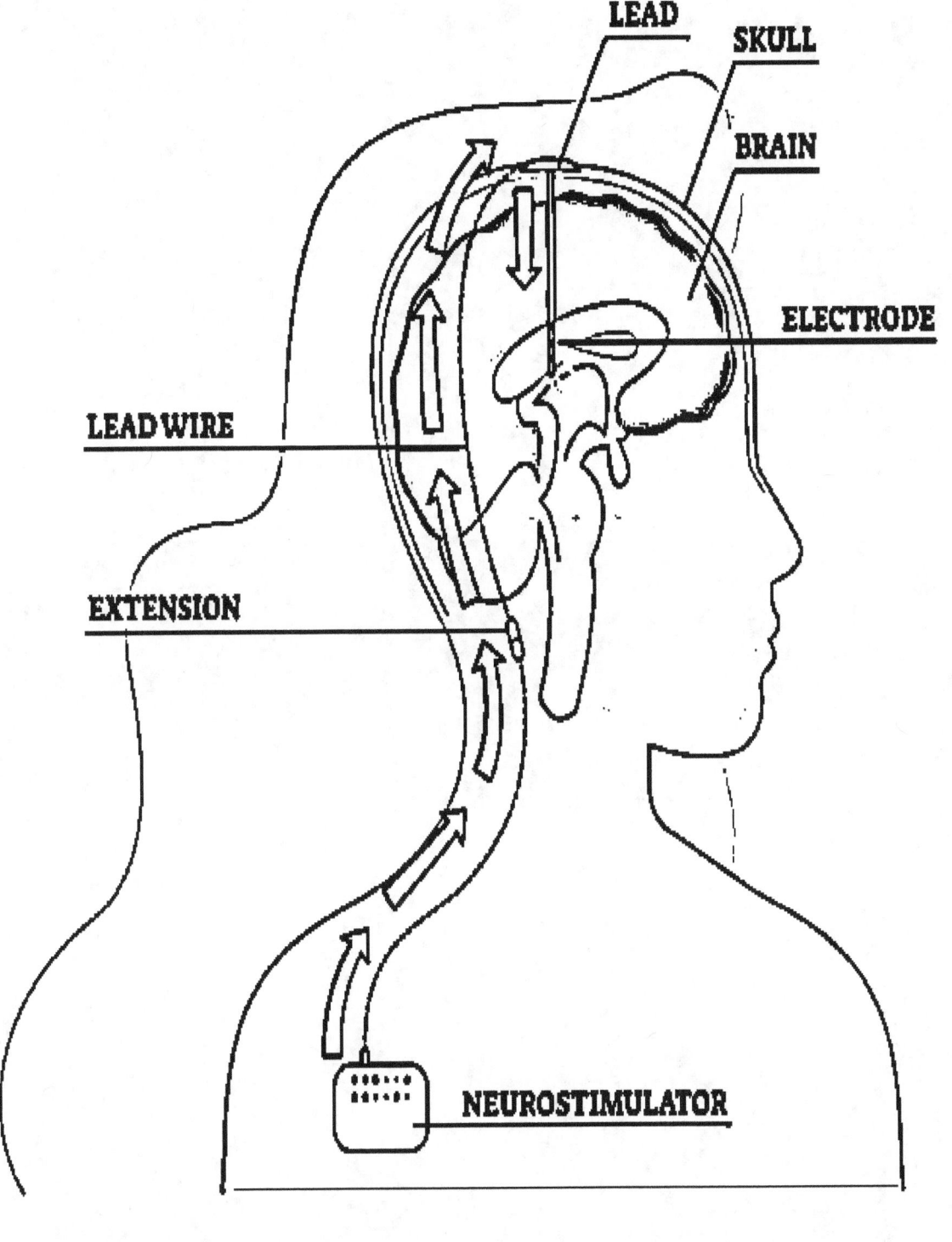

LEAD

SKULL

BRAIN

ELECTRODE

LEAD WIRE

EXTENSION

NEUROSTIMULATOR

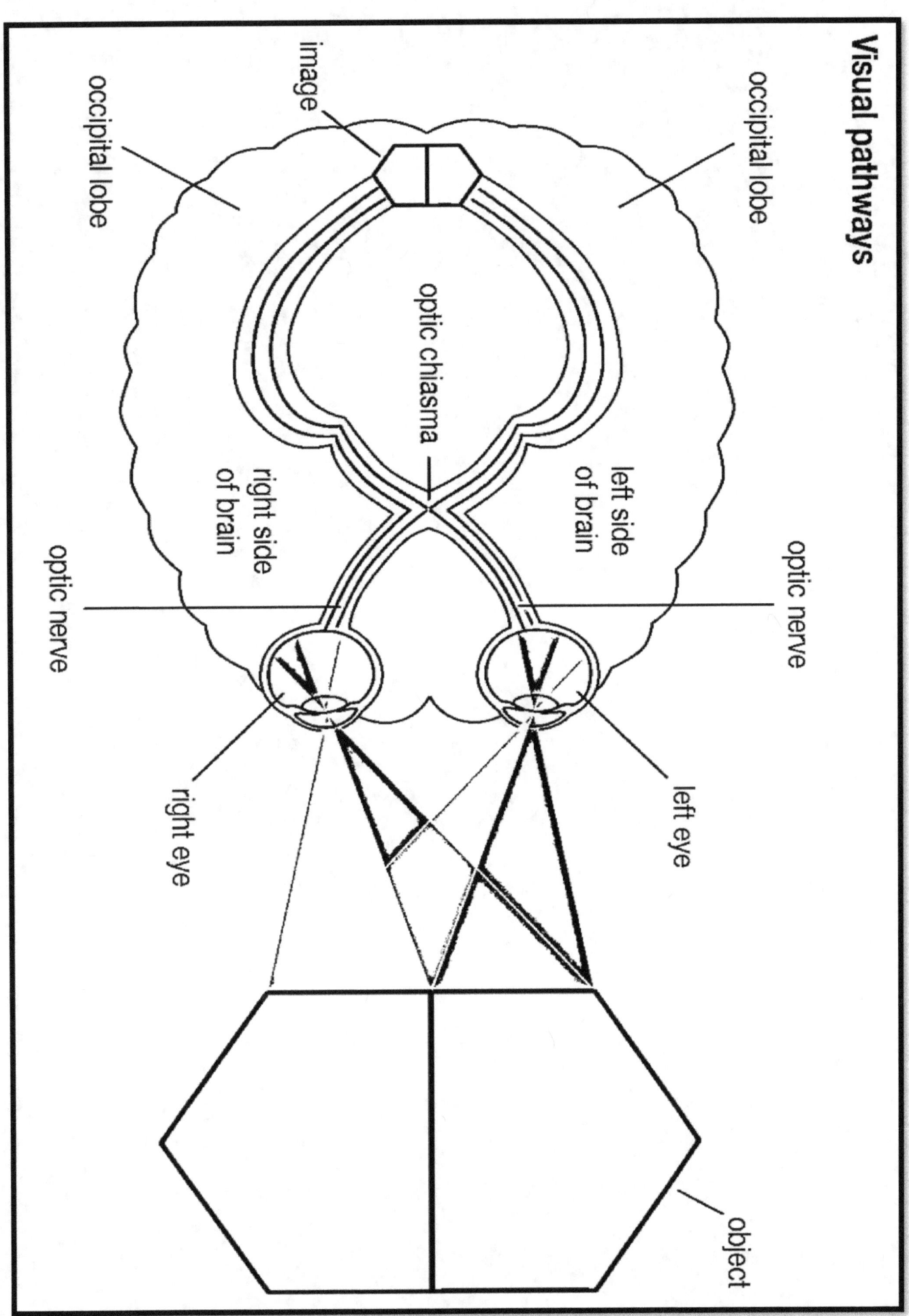

occipital lobe

occipital lobe

image

optic chiasma

right side
of brain

left side
of brain

optic nerve

optic nerve

right eye

left eye

object

Human Brain Anatomy

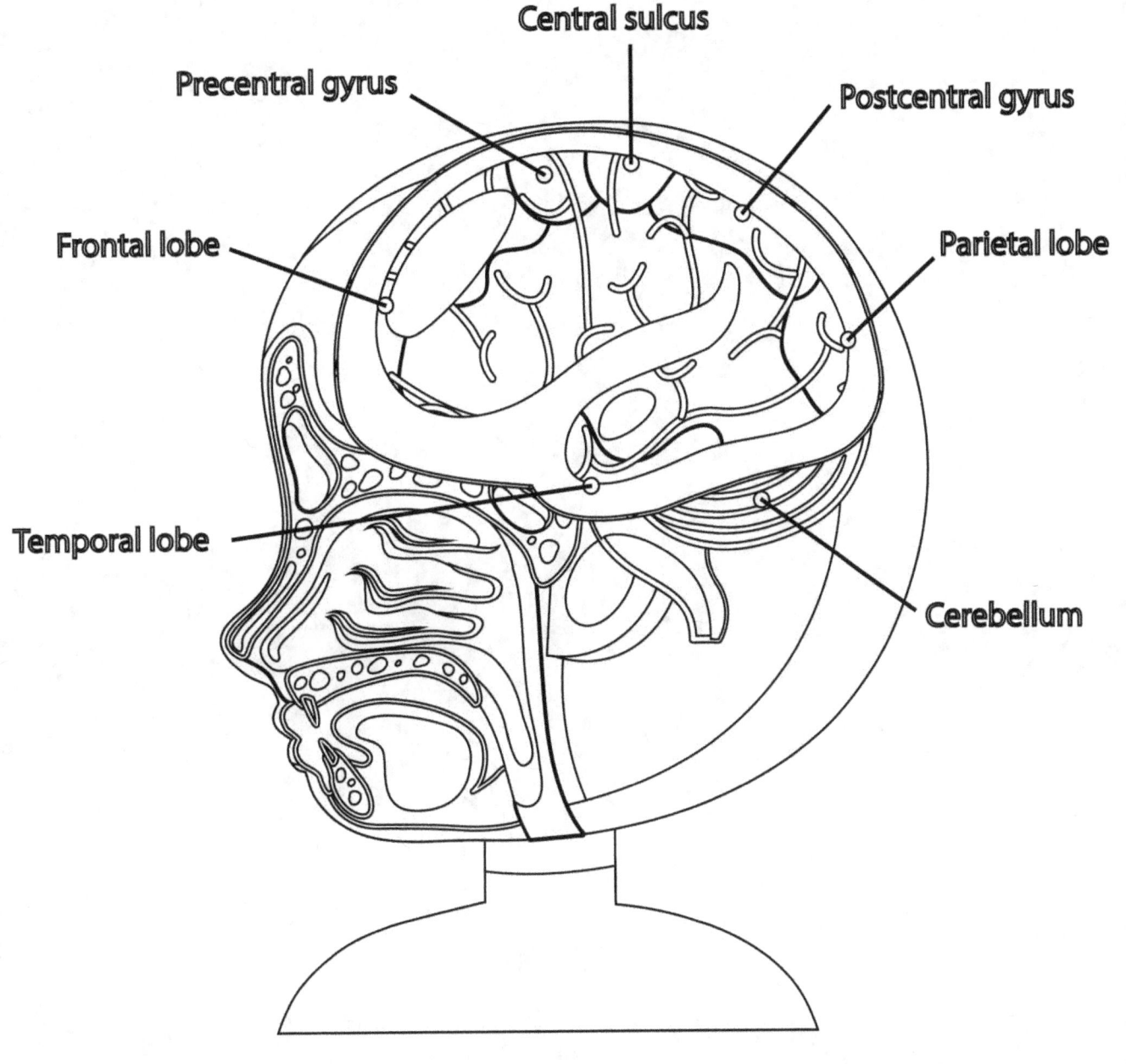

Central sulcus

Precentral gyrus

Postcentral gyrus

Frontal lobe

Parietal lobe

Temporal lobe

Cerebellum

BRAIN

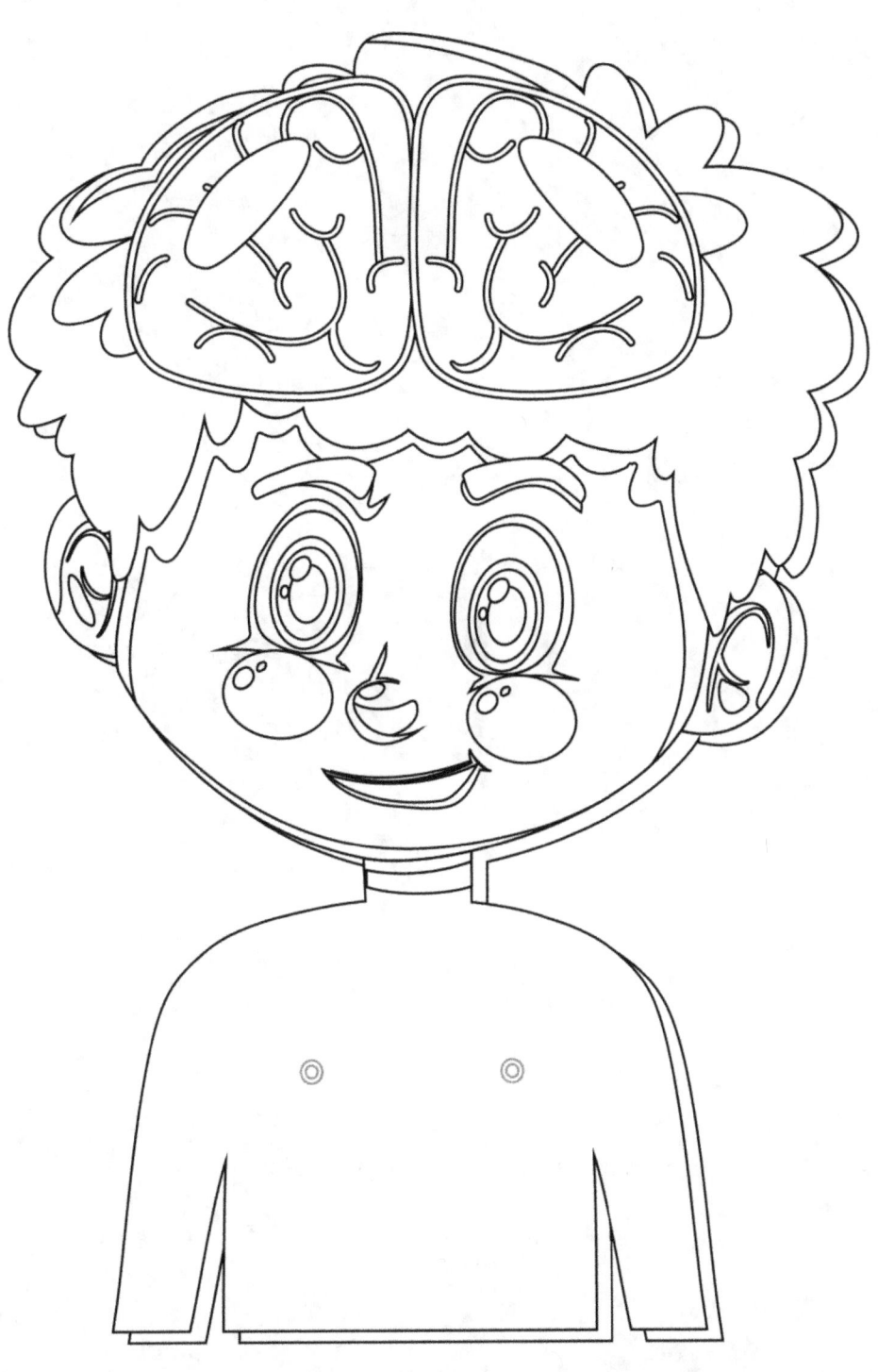

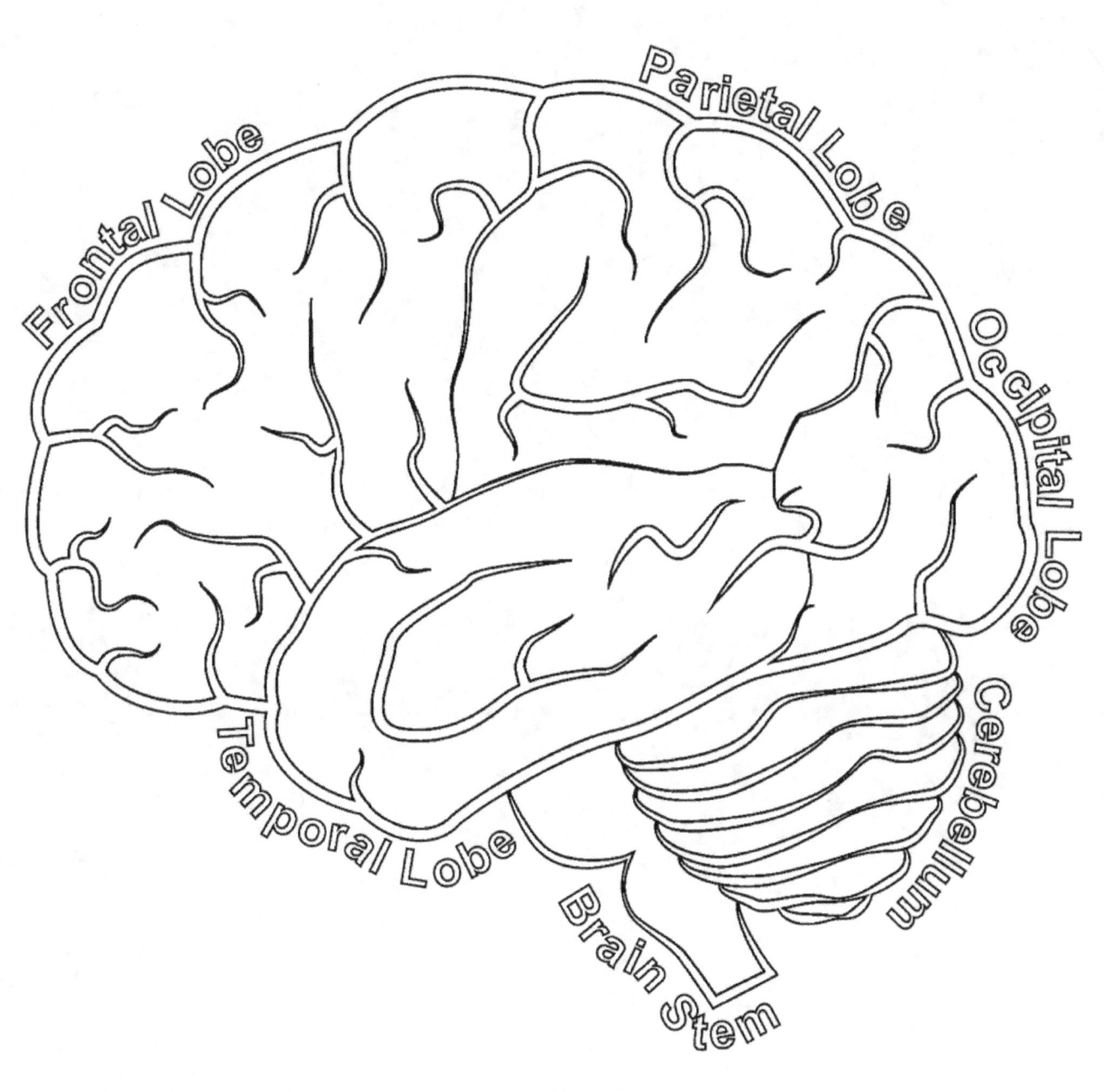

COLOUR EACH ZONE

LEFT BRAIN vs RIGHT BRAIN

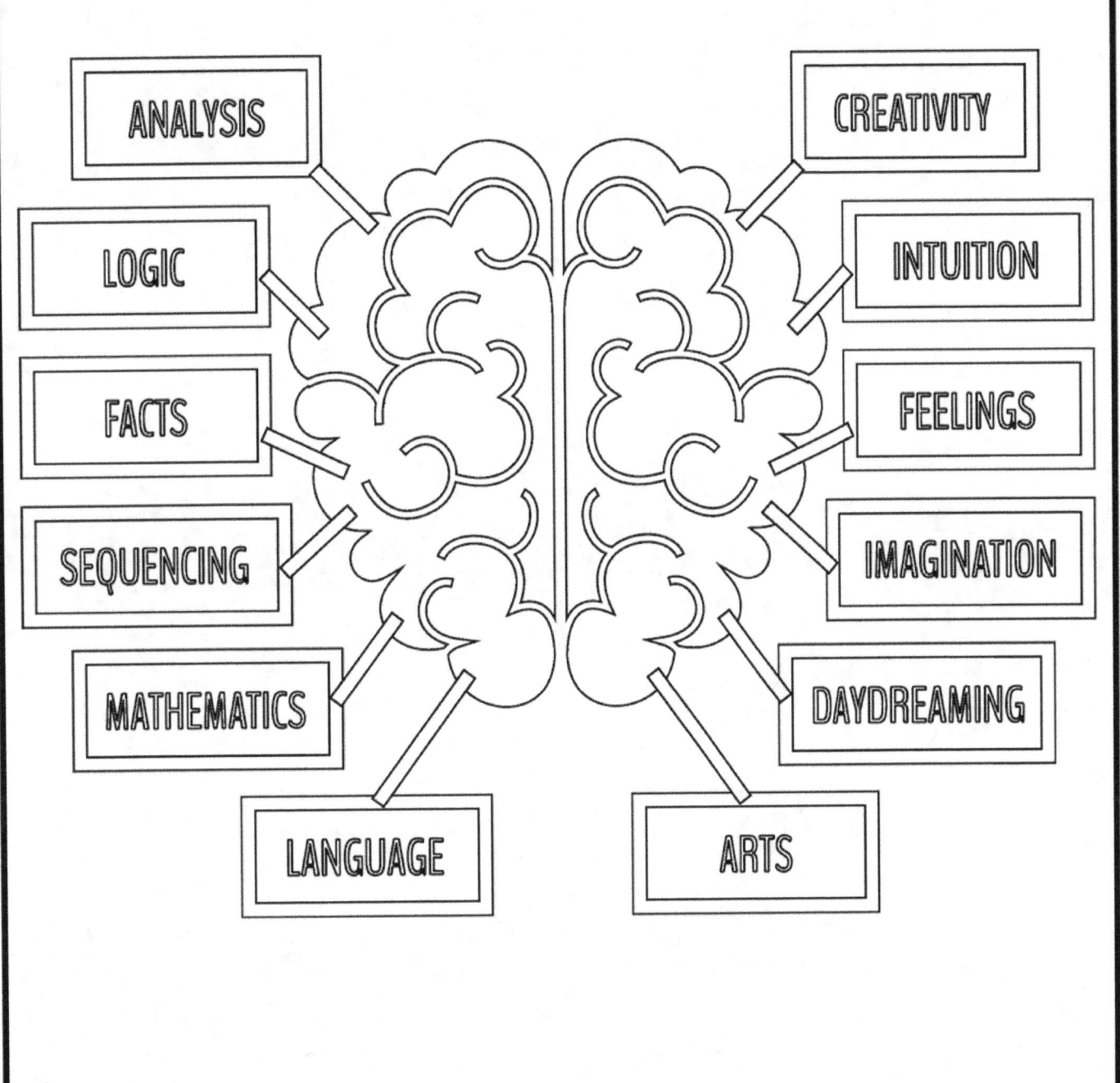

ANALYSIS

LOGIC

FACTS

SEQUENCING

MATHEMATICS

LANGUAGE

CREATIVITY

INTUITION

FEELINGS

IMAGINATION

DAYDREAMING

ARTS

CREATIVE BRAIN INFOGRAPHICS

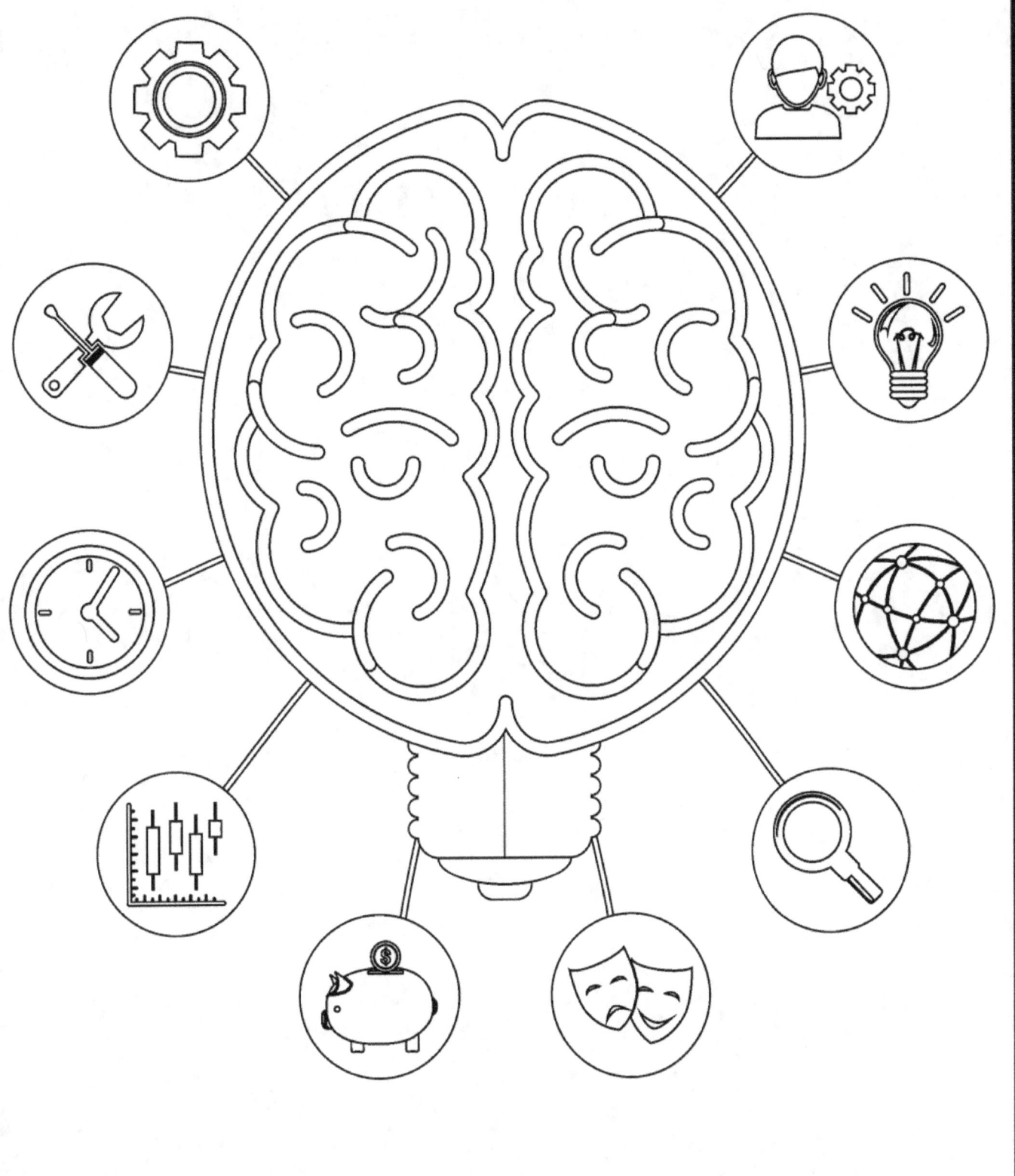

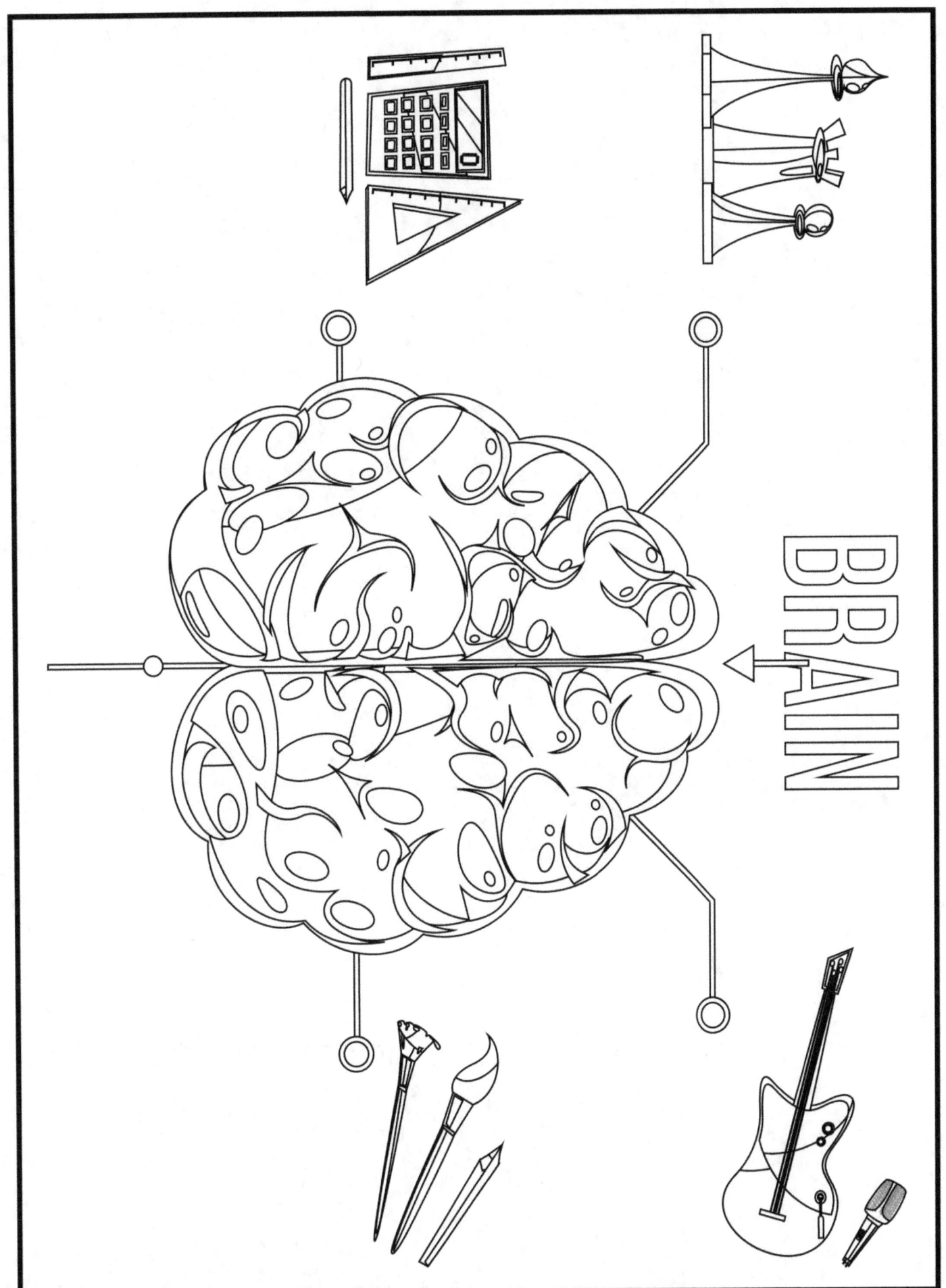

BRAIN

IF YOU ENJOY THIS BOOK , PLZ TAKE A FEW MINUTES TO LEAVE US A REVIEW ON AMAZON.

EACH ONE ON YOUR REVIEW IS REALY IMPORTANT TO BOST OUR WORK,

www.ingramcontent.com/pod-product-compliance
Lightning Source LLC
Chambersburg PA
CBHW081003290526
45795CB00009B/3054